GREEN TEA

FIGHT CANCER, LOWER CHOLESTEROL, LIVE LONGER

Kate Gilbert Udall

WOODLAND PUBLISHING

Pleasant Grove, UT

CONTENTS

GREEN TEA

INTRODUCTION

Only recently has the Western world discovered the benefits of drinking green tea that have been enjoyed by Asians for centuries. Though green tea has its origins in China, other Asian cultures have adopted green tea as a common drink and have reaped many health benefits. In Japan, for example, the custom of drinking green tea came from China about 1,100 years ago when Buddhist monks, who had gone to China for study, returned to Japan bringing tea with them as a medicinal beverage. The monk Eisai stressed the beneficial effects of tea in his book *Maintaining Health by Drinking Tea* (1211). He wrote:

> Tea is a miraculous medicine for the maintenance of health. Tea has an extraordinary power to prolong life. Anywhere a person cultivates tea, long life will follow. In ancient and modern times, tea is the elixir that creates the mountain-dwelling immortal.

Clearly, green tea has from early times been highly valued for its medicinal uses. And in recent years, research into the effects of green tea has progressed so far that scientific confirmation has been provided for the widespread belief that tea is key in the achievement and maintenance of good health. These studies are now confirming at least 4,000 years of folklore and medical practice in Asia regarding the incredible health benefits of green tea.

The many health benefits of tea, all of which have been demonstrated in scientific studies, include:

• Acting as a strong antioxidant
• Protecting against cancer
• Lowering cholesterol and blood pressure
• Working as antibacterial and antiviral agent
• Reducing blood sugar

Green tea may be the most valuable substance you can take to protect your general health. The major chemical component of the tea leaf that provides all these health benefits is a group of phytochemicals known as polyphenols.[1] Long known as tea tannin, and having an extremely pungent taste, polyphenols constitute 15 to 30 percent of dried green tea. In fresh tea leaves, these polyphenols exist as a series of chemicals called catechins, which include gallocatechin (GC), epigallocatechin (EGC), epicatechin (EC), epigallocatechin gallate (EGCg), and epicatechin gallate (Ecg). It's important to note that green tea is highest in EGCg, which most responsible for antioxidant activity. Green tea is also processed in a way that protects polyphenols by destroying the enzyme that oxidizes them.[2] The following chart shows the breakdown of chemical compounds in tea leaves and outlines their potential health benefits.[3]

Fight Cancer, Lower Cholesterol, Live Longer

INGREDIENT	AMOUNT IN TEA LEAVES	BIOLOGICAL EFFECTS
Polyphenols, Catechins, and its oxidated derivative	10-25%	Prevents oxidation/mutation, anticarcinogenic, lowers cholesterol level, lowers level of LDL in bloodstream, retards blood pressure increase, retards coagulation of red blood cells, antibiotic, prevents allergies, improves viral digestion in the intestines, eliminates body odor.
Flavonols	0.6-0.7%	Increases immunity of blood vessels, prevents oxidation, lowers blood pressure, eliminates body odor.
Caffeine	2-4%	Excites central nervous system, diuretic, prevents asthma, increases metabolic rate.
Complex sugars (Glycosides)	0.6%	Prevents increase in blood sugar.
Vitamin C	150-250 mg	Prevents oxidation, anticancer.
Vitamin E	25-70 mg	Prevents oxidation, anticarcinogenic, prevents infertility.
Carotene	13-29 mg	Prevents oxidation, anticarcinogenic, increases immunity.
Saponia	0.1%	Anticarcinogenic, prevents inflammation.
Flouride	90-350 PPM	Prevents cavities.
Zinc	30-75 PPM	Prevents skin inflammation, maintains level of immunity.
Selenium	1.0-1.8 PPM	Prevents oxidation, anticarcinogenic, prevents deterioration of the heart muscle.
Magnesia	400-2000 PPM	Prevents oxidation, increases immunity, assists in digestion of ethyl.

As the chart above illustrates, the health benefits of green tea are numerous and far-reaching. The remainder of this booklet will outline those benefits and present the most recent research supporting the health claims of green tea advocates. However, this guide is not a substitute for the advice of a physician. If you have health concerns, it is recommended that you seek medical counsel.

GREEN TEA AS AN ANTIOXIDANT

Though oxygen is necessary for human life, it can be a harmful agent in the form of active or free radical oxygen. Active oxygen is a problem because it can combine with anything in the body and oxidize it with consequent destruction of cell membranes, damage to DNA, and oxidation of lipids (fats). All of these can lead to diseases like cancer. Active oxygen combines with lipids in the body to create lipid peroxide, or lipids with excessive oxygen, which is a very harmful substance. Thus it is necessary for us to provide our bodies with something that can counter this activity—some form of antitoxin or antioxidant.

The antioxidant part of green tea has been shown to efficiently scavenge these toxins. In a study comparing the antioxidant effects of green tea and black tea, green tea was found to be six times more potent. Green tea's antioxidant activity is particularly important for preventing lipid peroxidation, which often plays a key role in the buildup of atherosclerotic plaque. Since lipid peroxidation is also a factor in the spoilage of oils and fatty constituents of many foods, the antioxidant ingredient in green tea helps prevent this spoilage.[4]

In experimental studies the polyphenols in green have actually shown greater antioxidant protection than well-known antioxidants vitamins C and E. And, in addition to exerting antioxidant activity on its own, green tea has been shown to increase the activity of the body's own antioxidant system, including activation of enzymes like superoxide dismutase and glutathione peroxidase.[5] Dennis Picard, ND, in a study of the make-up of green tea also notes that the antioxidation properties of green tea have been shown to effectively fight skin cancer. He reports:

> Green tea contains many polyphenol substances with exceptional antioxidant activity, and is consumed widely throughout the world. Green tea aqueous extract and its polyphenols, of which epigallocatechin gallate (EGCg) predominates, have been studied extensively in animal models for their antineplastic properties. EGCg and green tea olyphenols have been shown to inhibit skin tumor initiation, promotion and progression by a number of mechanisms . . .[6]

Picard goes on to advocate consuming green tea, saying, "It is evident that the consumption of green tea is beneficial in the prevention of cancer in these models."[7] Clearly, green tea can effectively work as an antioxidant agent and help to cleanse toxins from the body.

CANCER PREVENTION WITH GREEN TEA

Both green and black tea come from the leaves of the same plant, the tea plant (*Camelia sinensis*). The tea plant originated in China, but is now grown and consumed all over the world. Michael Murray, N.D., explains:

Green tea is produced by lightly steaming the fresh-cut black tea leaf; to produce black tea, the leaves are oxidized. During oxidation, many of the polyphenol substances, compounds with potent antioxidant and anticancer properties, are destroyed. Unlike black tea, green tea is very high in polyphenols.[8]

The anticancer effects are the result of the green-tea polyphenols blocking the formation of cancer-causing compounds as well as effectively detoxifying or trapping cancer-causing chemicals. Green tea polyphenols have shown greater antioxidant protection than have vitamins C and E in experimental studies. And, in addition to exerting antioxidant activity on its own, green tea has been shown to increase the activity of the body's own antioxidant system, including activation of enzymes like superoxide dismutase and glutathione peroxidase.[9]

The forms of cancer which appear to be prevented best by green tea are cancers of the gastrointestinal tract, including cancers of the stomach, small intestine, pancreas, and colon; lung cancer: and estrogen-related cancers, including most breast cancers. The popular custom of drinking green tea with meals is thought to be a major reason for the low rates of these cancers in Japan, for example. "With the cancer rate in the US rising, especially for these cancers where green tea has been shown to be protective, more Americans might want to start drinking green tea with their meals or taking a green-tea supplement."[10]

A report from the National Cancer Institute found that Chinese men and women who drink green tea have a reduced risk of developing esophageal skin cancer.[11] The researchers used a cancer registry to identify 902 esophageal cancer patients from urban Shanghai, People's Republic of China. This esophageal cancer study is part of a larger, multisite study that included pancreatic, colon, and rectal cancers.

"This is the first epidemiologic study to demonstrate that green tea may protect against esophageal cancer in humans," said Joseph McLaughlin, Ph. D., the lead researcher from NCI in the report. Animal studies have shown that green tea infusions and extracts protect against esophageal cancer, but this study is the first investigation involving humans to support the experimental evidence, Dr. McLaughlin also explained.

Patients ages 30 to 74 years who were diagnosed with esophageal cancer between October 1990 and January 1993 were interviewed on their residential and medical history, height, weight, diet, smoking habits, alcohol use, tea consumption, family history of cancer, occupation, physical activity, and reproductive history. There were 1,552 people without the disease (control subjects) who answered the same questions.

Information about tea consumption included types of tea consumed, frequency of consumption, and age at which tea drinking began. Researchers measured consumption in grams of tea leaves consumed per month. A tea drinker was defined as someone who drank at least one cup of tea per week for six months or longer. The study found that drinking green tea was associated with a 50 percent lower risk of esophageal cancer in women. Among men, risk was also reduced, but this finding was not statistically significant. However, green tea was linked to a 60 percent reduction of esophageal cancer among both men and women who did not smoke.[12]

These scientists support the claim that the protective effects of green tea arise out of polyphenol compounds in the tea. As stated previously, polyphenols have strong antioxidant properties and the ability to halt enzymes that produce carcinogens and the ability to inhibit cancer cell growth. According to Dr. McLaughlin, additional epidemiologic studies are needed to confirm the findings from this research. Should they be confirmed, Dr. McLaughlin believes that clinical trials should be undertaken to determine the preventative effects of green tea. These trials would allow researchers to better understand the biochemical mechanisms involved in the inhibition of esophageal cancer and to determine whether green tea can truly prevent its occurrence.

These findings are particularly important because in one year about 11,000 Americans will be diagnosed with esophageal cancer and 10,400 people will die of the disease.

Another report from the NCI, published by Reuters Health Information Services[13], reveals that an ingredient in green tea fights skin, lymph, and prostate cancers. Tests of the ingredient, EGCg, showed it killed cancer cells of skin, lymph system, and prostate tissue taken from both humans and mice while leaving healthy cells unharmed, report researchers from Case Western Reserve University.[14]

Exactly how the ingredient works against cancer remains unclear, says Dr. Hasan Mukhtar, senior study author and professor of dermatology at the university. But he notes that the compound leads to the programmed cell death, or apoptosis of cancer cells.[15] He says:

> It seems that somehow, through a cell-signaling pathway, it is communicated to the cancer cells that they better commit suicide or they'll be murdered, So cells make a decision and undergo apoptosis. And we don't know the signaling pathway.

Mukhtar goes on to say that evidence of apoptosis showed up as "very distinct, clear-cut features in the shape of the cells" and in the breakdown of their molecular structure. At the highest dose of the green tea ingredient, nearly all cells were found to be in the latest stage of apoptosis. These new findings add to previous test-tube studies showing that the tea ingredient prevented tumors in animal tissue. Dietary studies of tea consumption in people also suggest that green tea has some cancer preventive properties.

Some nutritional epidemiology studies have suggested that green tea consumption might be effective in the prevention of certain human cancers—cancers of the bladder, prostate, esophagus, and stomach, Mukhtar postulates. "For example, one hospital in Shanghai reported that the recurrence of esophageal cancer was low in that part of the population that was drinking green tea."

A cup of green tea contains between 100 and 200 milligrams of the anti-tumor ingredient, EGCg. Mukhtar and his associates advocate drinking green tea daily. They say, "Based on our studies and others, it seems four cups of green tea per day should be sufficient." They conclude that these findings warrant clinical trials on the green tea ingredient for people at high risk for cancer.

Similar studies have demonstrated protection against cancers of the esophagus, stomach, skin, breast, pancreas, colon/rectum and liver and others in tea-drinking humans and in animals fed green tea. For example, one study compared the frequency of a particular marker of lung cancer, the degradation of lymphocytes, in smokers and non-smokers. The marker was found to be significantly elevated in smokers who did not drink green tea, whereas, in those who drank green tea, the frequency was comparable to that of non-smokers.[16] And when mice were exposed to the carcinogens in cigarette smoke, those fed green tea extract had 45 percent lower incidence of lung cancer than their controlled counterparts.[17]

OTHER ENLIGHTENING FINDINGS

Numerous population-based studies have demonstrated that green tea consumption is associated with a significantly lower risk for many types of cancer. In addition to the population-based evidence, green tea and green-tea extracts have been shown to exert many anticancer effects in experimental studies.

Population-Based Research

Cancer mortality statistics on Japanese people indicate that the death rate from cancer is significantly lower, for both men and women, in areas (Shizuoka Prefecture is particularly noted) devoted to green tea production. In these regions there was a significantly lower death rate for all types of cancer in general and for gastrointestinal cancers such as stomach, esophagus and liver cancers in particular.[18] Further study showed that residents of these areas where green tea is a staple crop tend to drink the tea daily in strong concentrations.[19] It would seem from these results that green tea is connected in some way with cancer prevention.

Experimental-Based Research

In one experimental study mice were inoculated with cancer cells and then studied for the growth of malignancies. One group was given an extract of green tea while another group was not. Comparison of the two groups showed a marked reduction in the growth of tumors among those receiving the green tea.[20]

In further research, Professor Shu-Jun Cheng of the Cancer Institute, Chinese Academy of Medical Science in Beijing and Dr. Ito Oguni gave mice substances which, when transformed in the body to cancer-causing chemicals, generate carcinoma in both the esophagus and stomach. The researchers then proceeded to check if green tea had the ability to inhibit the development of these cancers. Administration of green tea did indeed reduce the incidence of cancer to less that 50 percent.[21]

The underlying generation of cancer is not completely understood but involves at least two stages. A substance capable of causing mutations (initiator) first damages DNA in the cell and renders it subject to cancer (initiation). This condition then remains unchanged for some time until another substance, which activates cancer (promoter) leads to the actual growth of a malignancy (promotion).[22] Although the cause of cancer is not understood, it is clear from recent research that extract of green tea and catechin can markedly inhibit both stages of cancer development.[23]

Cholesterol Reduction

Cholesterol is usually cited as the "bad guy" for causing various diseases in adults, but it is a chemical present in all animals and necessary in our bodies for important processes such as manufacturing cell membranes and fusing cells. There are two types of cholesterol: one is the cholesterol (LDL- and VLDL-cholesterol), often referred to as "bad," that accumulates in tissues and the other is the "good" cholesterol (HDL-cholesterol) that collects excessive cholesterol from the tissues. If the amount of bad cholesterol in the blood becomes too much, it is collected on blood vessel walls and can lead to atherscloerosis. Atherscloerosis in conjunction with high blood pressure can cause myocardial infarction and cerebral infarction. Good cholesterol, however, can prevent atherscloerosis and should exist in proper balance for good health.

Studies in animals have revealed a significant and necessary action of green tea. In one study, rats were fed a fat-enriched diet for 28 days; the diet of some of the animals was also supplemented with green tea. Those rats fed the tea extract showed significant reductions in plasma total cholesterol, VLDL- and LDL-cholesterol ("bad"), and increases in HDL-cholesterol ("good"). The green tea catechin restricts the excessive buildup of blood cholesterol.[24]

In another experiment rats were fed a high-fat, high-cholesterol diet. After four weeks, the total cholesterol level in the group that did not receive the EGCg rose to more than twice that of the control group. In those rats fed a diet containing 1.0 percent EGCg, this effect was even more pronounced. These results suggest that hyperlipidemia—excessive cholesterol in the lipids—can be controlled to a large degree simply by ingesting a green tea extract containing EGCg.

Humans seem to experience a similar effect. In a study of more than 2000 Japanese men aged 49 to 55, tea consumption (10 cups/day) was found to significantly lower serum levels of total cholesterol and LDL-cholesterol, but did not seem to affect levels of HDL-cholesterol or triglycerides.[25]

Blood Pressure Reduction

High blood pressure is known to give the vascular system serious problems and contributes to atherscloerosis. Atherscloerosis will then initiate heart disease, stroke, and other cardiovascular diseases. The cause of high blood pressure is not yet fully understood, but it is known that a chemical called angiotensin II plays a role in high blood pressure.

In hypertension caused by high blood pressure, angiotensin I converting enzyme (ACE) converts angiotensin I to vasoconstrictive angiotensin II. When this process is blocked, it is possible to prevent hypertension to a large extent. This is the mechanism that ACE-inhibitor drugs use to treat high blood pressure.

There are, however, other effective means to treat high blood pressure. Green tea polyphenols also have significant ACE-inhibiting ability. In one study, tea polyphenols were given to a group of genetically hypertensive rats beginning one week after weaning; a second group received a normal diet. After 16 weeks, the diets were switched. The blood pressure in the normal diet group already exceeded a very high level at 10 weeks, compared with no clear rise in blood pressure in the tea polyphenol-treated group. When the diets were switched at 16 weeks, the blood pressure changed accordingly. The researchers also found that the hypertensive rats on a normal diet were more likely to die of a stroke.[26]

GREEN TEA'S ANTIBACTERIAL AND ANTIVIRAL ACTIVITY

Tea catechins are strong antibacterial and antiviral agents which make them effective for treating everything from tooth decay to HIV. Studies show that tea catechins can protect mice against infection from the bacteria that cause cholera.[27] Green tea has been shown to inhibit the spread of *Clostridium spp*, which is associated with wide-ranging human diseases that result in sudden death, toxicity, mutagenesis, carcinogenesis, and aging.[28] And the polyphenols in green tea kill *Staphylococcus aureus* in the respiratory tract, a bacteria which has been shown to be resistant to methicillin—an antibody. Polyphenols were also shown in this study to make these bacteria more susceptible to oxacillin.[29]

The effect of green tea extract on viral infections is also remarkable. Japanese researchers have now shown that EGCg and other tea polyphenols prevent the influenza virus from adhesion to normal cells, thus blocking flu infection. Even a small amount of EGCg seems to be able to present a significant obstruction in the way of the flu virus.[30] Green tea has often been used as a remedy for diarrhea. Recent research has revealed why it works in treating diarrhea. Polyphenols act against infections caused by enterovirus, which are common causes of diarrhea.[31]

Perhaps the best-documented antimicrobial effect of tea catechins is against bacteria that cause tooth decay. In fact, green tea is probably better than fluoride for good oral hygiene. In one study, green tea was found to be far more effective against *S mutans*.[32] Another recent study found that EGCg completely inhibited the growth and cellular adherence of another important oral bacteria, *Porphyromonas gingivalis*.[33] It has been suggested that green tea be used as a preventive measure in root canals because of its broad spectrum of antibacterial activity.[34]

REDUCTION OF BLOOD SUGAR

About 60 years ago, Dr. Minowada of Kyoto University noticed that sugar in the urine of patients hospitalized for diabetes fell markedly during periods when they participated in chanoyu (Tea Ceremony). He reported that powdered tea of the type used in the traditional tea ceremony had the capability of lowering blood sugar.[35] Unfortunately, the outbreak of World War II and accompanying food shortages stole the attention warranted by this important discovery. But the "gourmet era" in recent years in Japan has led to new interest in diabetes and the ability of green tea to reduce blood sugar.

The sugars and carbohydrates in our food are digested mainly in the duodenum, converted there to glucose and then absorbed into the blood. The agent that regulates the intake of blood sugar into the tissues is insulin, a chemical secreted from the Langerhans islets on the pancreas. Diabetes is a disease characterized by insufficient secretion or improper functioning of insulin, which hinders the proper absorption of glucose into the tissues and leads to a high concentration of blood sugar that must be eventually excreted into the urine. In a recent study, mice subject to hereditary diabetes were given dried green tea catechin in edible form and experienced lower blood sugar.[36]

CONCLUSION

The health benefits of green tea are varied and wide-ranging. Because the chemical makeup of green tea gives it the capability to positively affect so many different systems of the human body, it makes sense to use it in achieving those health benefits. Now that science has begun to elucidate and confirm the benefits of specific agents in green tea, those interested in achieving or maintaining good health can use green tea to an even greater advantage. And for those who think that 4 to 10 cups of tea a day sounds like a little too much, green tea is currently available in a convenient supplement. What Asians have known for centuries about drinking green tea can now benefit the entire world.

ENDNOTES

1. Green tea extract. *http: //www.life-enhancement.com/n37/n37 greentea.html.*
2. Green tea extract. *http: //www.life-enhancement.com/n37/n37 greentea.html.*
3. Tea: Chemical Compounds In Tea Leaves and Their Health Benefits. *http: //www.tenren.com/at-chem.html.*
4. Green tea extract. *http: //www.life-enhancement.com/n37/n37 greentea.html*
5. Murray, Michael N.D. "Fighting cancer with a cup, or more, of green tea." *Better Nutrition.* (Jan. 1998).
6. Picard, Dennis. "The biochemistry of green tea polyphenols and their potential application in human skin cancer." *Alternative Medicine Review,* 1 (1996): 31-42.
7. Picard, Dennis. "The biochemistry of green tea polyphenols and their potential application in human skin cancer." *Alternative Medicine Review,* 1 (1996): 31-42.
8. Murray, Michael N.D. "Fighting cancer with a cup, or more, of green tea." *Better Nutrition.* (Jan. 1998).
9. Murray, Michael N.D. "Fighting cancer with a cup, or more, of green tea." *Better Nutrition.* (Jan. 1998).
10. Murray, Michael N.D. "Fighting cancer with a cup, or more, of green tea." *Better Nutrition.* (Jan. 1998).
11. "Study finds green tea may protect against esophageal cancer."*Cancernet: The National Cancer Institute http://www.graylab.ac. uk/cancernet/600411.htm*
12. Gao YT, McLaughlin JK, Blot WJ, et al. "Reduced risk of esophageal cancer associated with green tea consumption." *Journal of National Cancer Institute,* 86 (1994): 855-858.
13. "Green tea ingredient fights cancer." *Reuters Health Information Services http:// www.yahoo.com/headlines//health/stories/green_1*
14. Mukhtar, H. et al. *Journal of the National Cancer Institute,* 89 (1997):

1881-1886.

15. Mukhtar, H. et al. *Journal of the National Cancer Institute*, 89 (1997): 1881-1886.

16. Shim J, Kang M, Kim Y, Roh J, Roberts C, Lee I. "Chemoprotective effect of green tea (*Camellia sinensis*) among cigarette smokers." *Cancer Epidemiological Biomarkers Prevention*, 4 (1995): 387-391.

17. Brody, J. "Scientists seeking wonder drugs in tea." *The New York Times*. 14 March 1991. New York edition.

18. Oguni, I et al. *Japanese Journal of Nutrition*, 47 (1989): 31.

19. Oguni, I. *Metabolism and Disease*, 29 (1992): 453.

20. Oguni, I. *Biological Chemistry*, 52 (1988): 1879.

21. Oguni, Ito and Shu Jun Cheng. *Annual Report of the Skylark FoodScience Institute*. 3, (1991): 57.

22. "Green tea prevents cancer." *http: //www.daisan.co.jp./health2.htm.*

23. Nakamura et al. *PROC of International Tea-Quality—Human Health Symposium*, pp 227-38, (Hangzhou, China, Nov. 1987).

24. Muramatsu K, Fukuyo M, Hara Y. "Effect of green tea catechins on plasma cholesterol level in cholesterol-fed rats." *Journal of Nutritional Science Vitaminology*, 36 (1988): 227-233.

25. Kono S, Shinchi K, Wakabayashi K et al. "Relation of green tea consumption to serum lipids and lipid proteins in Japanese men." *Journal of Epidemiology*, 6 (1996), 128-133.

26. Hara Y, Matsuzaki T. and Suzuki T. Nippon Nogeikagaku Kaishi, 61 (1987): 803-10.

27. Toda M, Okubo S, Ilkigai H et al." The protective activity of tea catechins against experimental infection by vibrio cholerae 01." *Microbiol Immuniol*, 36 (1992): 999-1001.

28. Ahn Y-J, Kawamura T, Kim M, Yamamoto, T, Mitsuoka T. "Tea polyphenols: selective growth inhibitors of Clostridium spp." *Agric Biol Chem*, 55 (1991): 1425-1426.

29. Takahashi O, Cai Z, Toda M, Hara Y Shimamura T. "Appearance of antibacterial activity of oxacillin against methacillin-resistant Staphylococcus aureus (MRSA) in the presence of catechin." *Kansenshogaku Zasshi.*, 69 (1995): 1126-1134.

30. Nakayama M, Suzuki K, Toda M, Okubo S, Hara Y, Shimamura T. "Inhibition of the infectivity of influenza virus by tea polyphenols." *Antiviral Research*, 21 (1993): 289-299.

31. Mukoyama A, Ushijima H, Nishimura S et al. "Inhibition of rotavirus and enterovirus infections by tea extracts." *Jpn J Med Sci Biol*, 44 (1991): 181-186.

32. Sakanaka S, Kim M, Taniguchi M, Yamamoto T. "Antibactrial substances in Japanese green tea against Streptococcus mutans, a carcinogenic bacterium." *Agric Biol Chem*, 53 (1993): 2307-2311.

33. Sakanaka S, Aizawa M, Kim M, Yamamoto T. "Inhibitory effects of green tea polyphenols on growth and cellular adherence of an oral bacterium, Porphyromonas gingivalis." *Bioscience, Biotechnology, and Biochemistry*, 60 (1996): 745-49.

34. Horiba N, Ito M, Matsumoto T, Nakamura H. "A pilot study of Japanese green tea as a medicament: antibactrial and bactericidal effects." *Journal of Endodontics*, 17 (1991): 122-24.

35. "Green tea lowers the blood sugar level." *http: //www.daisan.co.jp/ health5.htm.*

36. Shimizu M et al. *Yakugaku Zasshi*, 108 (1988): 964.